Low GI Diet

C000152316

A Beginner's Step by Step Guide To Manage Weight Loss

Includes Recipes and a Meal Plan

mindplusfood

THANK YOU FOR YOUR PURCHASE

VISIT MINDPLUSFOOD.COM FOR A FREE 41-PAGE HOLISTIC HEALTH CHEAT SHEET

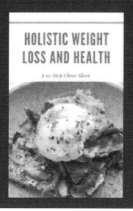

Table Of Contents

Disclaimer

By reading this disclaimer, you are accepting the terms of the disclaimer in full. If you disagree with this disclaimer, please do not read the book. The content in this book is provided for informational and educational purposes only.

This book is not intended to be a substitute for the original work of this diet plan. At most, this book is intended to be beginner's supplement to the original work for this diet plan and never act as a direct substitute. This book, is an overview, review, and commentary of the facts of that diet plan.

All product names, diet plans, or names used in this book are for identification purposes only and are property of their respective owners. Use of these names does not imply endorsement. All other trademarks cited herein are property of their respective owners.

None of the information in this book should be accepted as independent medical or other professional advice.

The information in the books has been compiled from various sources that are deemed reliable. It has been analyzed and summarized to the best of the Author's ability, knowledge, and belief. However, the Author cannot guarantee the accuracy and thus should not be held liable for any errors.

You acknowledge and agree that the Author of this book will not be held liable for any damages, costs, expenses, resulting from the application of the information in this book, whether directly or indirectly. You acknowledge and agree that you assume all risk and responsibility for any action you undertake in response to the information in this book.

You acknowledge and agree that by continuing to read this book, you will (where applicable, appropriate, or necessary) consult a qualified medical professional on this information. The information in this book is not intended to be any sort of medical advice and should not be used in lieu of any medical advice by a licensed and qualified medical professional.

Introduction

I want to thank you and congratulate you for getting this guide.

This guide is not about restricting yourself from eating the food that you love. It is not about losing weight drastically. This is not like other diet plans where you have to bust your pockets just to follow the strict regimen.

This book will teach you to choose and eat the right kind of food groups to lose weight. This is about getting a balanced diet that results in a healthy body by keeping your blood sugar level down.

From this book, you'll learn how to manage your weight by following the Low Glycemic Diet Plan. This is not a fad diet, like the most popular diet menu plans. This actually facilitates a change in your eating habit that you can eventually incorporate into your lifestyle.

In this book, I will introduce to you the concept of Low Glycemic Diet and share with you a sample meal plan and recipe that you can use as a starter.

I will walk with you as you start a new habit that will change your perception about eating and dieting.

Thanks again for getting this guide. I hope you enjoy it!

Chapter 1- Carbohydrates and the Glycemic Index

Before we get into Low Glycemic Diet, let's discuss what Low Glycemic Index or GLI is. In glycemic index, numbers are assigned to different food groups that contain carbohydrates. It is also indicative on a particular food's impact on your blood sugar level. The glycemic index in itself is not a diet plan but a tool that helps you count carbohydrates in your food choices.

Counting Carbohydrates

The carbohydrates in food are broken down into glucose and insulin, to be distributed to your body through the bloodstream.

Depending on how much carbohydrates you consumed and physical activities, these sugars will be converted to calories or will be stored in the body as fat reserves.

However, not all carbohydrates are sugar. Carbohydrates also come in the form of starchy and fibrous foods. Among the three, fiber is the only one that does not contain glucose and does not provide energy directly to your body. Fiber feeds the bacteria in your digestive system to produce fatty acids that your body can use as energy.

The glycemic index was designed to count carbohydrates in all of its different forms.

The Glycemic Index

Canadian scientist, David Jenkins, developed the Glycemic Index in 1981. He developed the GI as a dietary management tool for type 1 diabetes. The GI is an alternative way to classify carbohydrates. The study revolves around 62 commonly eaten carbo-loaded foods and the impact it has on blood sugar levels.

From this study came the glycemic index ranking:

>Low: 0 – 55
>Medium: 56 – 69
>High: 70 or more

The index preference is the Low GI value as food is digested and absorbed slowly thus, causing smaller and slower increase in blood sugar level.

In contrast, food with high GI value should be least preference because they are digested and absorbed faster, causing a rapid increase in blood sugar level.

The Glycemic Load Rating

The three factors affecting how fast food can increase your blood sugar are:

- *type of carbohydrate*
- *nutrient composition*
- *amount of food intake*

The GI does not take into account the amount of food eaten and to solve this, they developed the glycemic load rating (GL rating). GL takes into consideration the glycemic index and the grams per serving of the food you take.

The GL ranking has three classifications:
Low: 0 – 10
Medium: 11 – 19
High: 20 or more

The recommended total daily GL is no more than 100. You can calculate the Glycemic load (GL) as: *carbohydrate content x GI value / 100*

Example: cabbage has GI value of 10 and carbo content of 5.9 g. Following the equation: 5.9 g x 10/100 = 0.59. The Glycemic load of cabbage is <1 which is with the low value range.
If you wish to find the GI and GL of common foods, you can check out this **index list**.

Benefits of Using Glycemic Index

Carbohydrates is one of the three major macronutrients that the body needs. You cannot leave it out of your meal plan. The human body needs macronutrients to function properly.

The main purpose of using the glycemic index as part of your eating habit is to be able to choose the right kind of carbo-loaded food that will not cause a rapid increase in your blood sugar level.

Although the main purpose is to control a person's sugar level, the use of glycemic index has given additional benefits to its users.

- The use of low GI can help lower cholesterol level, particularly bad cholesterol or LDL. The increase of dietary fiber from fruits, vegetables, and whole grains can help lower overall cholesterol level.

- Low GI diet delays feelings of hunger due to slow increase of blood sugar and insulin response. The long-term result is gradual weight loss and better weight management.

- Helps control diabetes. One of the hardest thing for a diabetic to control is their blood sugar level. Almost every food available has carbohydrates. Using the low GI diet not only helps limit your carbohydrates, it also helps identify which type of food has more fiber than glucose.

- Helps minimize heart disease. Using low GI diet helps control increase of cholesterol. Cholesterol can cause high blood pressure and ultimately heart disease.

Now that you know more about Low Glycemic Index and how it works, allow me to walk you through the step-by-step guide on starting your own LGI diet.
I have designed a 3-week guide that you can use to start the Low Glycemic Index Diet and making it your new eating habit.

Chapter 2 Week 1: Getting Started

The first week is the preparation week. Before we start, let's do some pre-LGI diet check and preparation.

You can incorporate the low glycemic diet program with your current diet regimen. If your doctor or nutritionist prescribed a diet regimen for you, there is no need to change it.

Keep in mind that low glycemic diet is not about dieting. It is making smart food choices that will help lower your blood sugar levels.

Your meal should still be within the context of your prescribed diet. It is best to consult your physician or nutritionist before embarking on this diet.

Week 1
1. List down your current diet / current food list

List down the ingredients of the food you eat whether you are using a prescribed diet or not. Based on these ingredients, check the low glycemic index if the ingredients are within the allowable value of a low glycemic diet.
2. Compare your list against the list of what is approved as low glycemic food

Compare the carbohydrates count of your food ingredients against that low glycemic index. You can get the **index list** online.

As you have learned earlier, the acceptable index for low glycemic is 0-55. When you compare the list, you have to mark the ingredients that have an index number more than 55.

There are food groups that do not contain GI value because they have very little or no carbohydrates. You can add the following foods as part of your low GI diet:

- Meat: beef, pork, chicken, lamb and eggs
- Seafoods and Fish: examples are salmon, tuna, trout, sardines, and prawns
- Fats and Oils: examples are olive oil, butter, margarine, rice bran oil
- Nuts: examples are cashews, almonds, walnuts, pistachios, and macadamia
- Herbs and Spices: like salt, pepper, basil, dill, and garlic

If there are items you cannot find in the list, you can check out other sources like the **Health Harvard Glycemic Index Listing** and the **Glycemic Index Food Listing**.

3. Find alternative food for high value numbers

After comparison, you are likely to find food that will not fall on the low glycemic index. No need to worry. You can substitute them with other food groups. In Chapter 1 we discussed that not all carbohydrates comes from sugar and not all carbohydrates give high sugar content.

Example the index value of ice cream is 51 you can substitute it with fruit yogurt, which only has an index of 41. Although ice cream falls in the allowable low glycemic value, substituting it with yogurt will give you a much lower value.

4. Finalizing your list

Finalize your list. Do not choose food items randomly just because they are within the low glycemic level.
You are going to eat this food, so you have to be able to enjoy it. If you are not fond of eating apples (GI=36), don't force yourself. Replace it with something you can actually eat like oranges (GI=43).
If you are lactose intolerant, don't drink milk. You can drink soymilk instead.
Again, you have to keep in mind that you are not under a strict diet (unless you are under a prescribed diet). The Low Glycemic Diet has only one rule, choose the food that will not increase your blood sugar level and within an acceptable glycemic load.

Chapter 3 Week 2: Creating Your Meal Plan

A meal plan is a calendar of the food you are allowed to consume during every meal. A meal consists of breakfast, morning snack, lunch, afternoon snack, dinner, and nighttime snack (optional).

You can prepare a 7-day meal plan, or a 14-day meal plan or even a 30-day meal plan. It all depends on you.

For this exercise, we will prepare a 5-day meal plan. The short-term meal plan allows you to make adjustments easily. This is your first meal plan and you cannot rush the process.

Your body needs to adjust to your new eating habits slowly. Often, with fad diets, the adjustment is drastic. This does not allow your body to adjust to the changes, thus you end up cheating or giving up the diet.

Week 2

1. ## Creating your recipes

You'll find many low glycemic recipes that you can find online. You can also use non-low glycemic recipes and substitute the ingredients with low glycemic alternatives.

2. ## Checking the calories and macronutrients count

The USDA Dietary Guidelines, standard daily calorie is 2,000 calories to maintain and 1,500 calories to lose one pound of weight every week. However, this would depend on other factors like age, height, activity levels, current weight, metabolic health and others.

Most recipes currently available in the net includes calorie count and macronutrients count. You can easily get the GI for each ingredient and check the total Glycemic Load based on the calorie count per serving of each recipe.

Remember the equation of the GL in Chapter 1. Use that to check the GL of your recipe. Although the glycemic index is still the deciding factor for low glycemic diet, it is still recommended to monitor the glycemic load of your food intake.

3. ## Make your shopping list

Once you have your recipes, time to do the shopping.

You actually don't have to make a big change when doing your shopping. The difference now is you will have to choose food group and ingredients that have low glycemic reading.

You simply cannot pick up all the food you *want*.

Before you go to the grocery store, list down the ingredients for all your recipes. There is a big chance that some of the ingredients are the same in different recipes so you can save yourself some money by buying them in bulk.

It is better to do your shopping before you finalize your meal plan because you might find that some ingredients that are not available. This way, you will finalize your meal plan based on the available ingredients rather than going crazy finding the ingredients to fit your meal plan, which can be costly and time consuming.

When doing your grocery, there are ingredients that you might have to buy in can or processed. There's really no way to know the glycemic value of canned or processed food but here a few tips:

- Check the ratio of the carbohydrates content versus the protein and fats. If the carbohydrates ratio is lower, then chances are the product is low glycemic.

- Take note that the word total carbohydrates in food labels often refers to starch and sugars. The fiber content is removed during processing leaving just the sugar and starch.
- Any food, especially soluble food that has high fiber content is usually has low glycemic index value.
- Food with low glycemic value bears the GI symbol is guarantee that the food is low glycemic.

4. Create your meal plan

So now, it's time to create your meal plan. As mentioned, for this exercise we will start with a 5-day meal plan consisting of breakfast, lunch, dinner and two snacks.
If you have a prescribed meal plan, stick with it. Just substitute the food items or ingredients with a low glycemic value.

5-day Meal Plan

	Breakfast	Snack	Lunch	Snack	Dinner
Day 1	1 bowl **Quinoa and black beans** 2 slices low sodium bacon ½ cup Orange Juice	1 mozzarella cheese stick 8 oz. water	1 halve side **Crab Stuff Avocado** 2 slices toast wheat bread 1 small peach 8 oz. water	1 cup fruit salad (kiwi, apple, orange, grapefruit) 8 oz. water	1 serving **Lemon Chicken Salad** 1 slice barley bread 8 oz. water
Day 2	½ cup Quinoa Porridge with ½ cup raspberries 2 slices turkey bacon 8 oz. coffee with almond milk	6 almond flour cracker 1 tbsp. peanut butter 8 oz. water	**Beef Stew** 2 slices rye bread 1 pear 8 oz. water	1 almond muffin 8 oz. water	**Tomato & Basil Soup** 1 cup steamed cauliflower 8 oz. water
Day 3	1 bowl apple muesli 2 poached egg 8 oz. unsweetened iced tea	6 oz. yogurt ½ cup strawberries 8 oz. water	**Grilled tenderloin** ½ cup mix lettuce, onion, tomato w/ vinaigrette 1 small apple 8 oz. water	8 oz. protein shake 8 oz. water	1 bowl mixed green salad w/ apple cider 1 slice grilled salmon w/ lemon 8 oz. water
Day 4	1 piece buckwheat pancake w/ blueberries 2 boiled eggs ½ large grapefruit 8 oz. coffee with skim milk and stevia	2 slices cinnamon and almond loaf 8 oz. water	**Braised balsamic chicken** 2 slices wheat bread ½ cup strawberries 8 oz. water	1 tub Greek yogurt 8 oz. water	1 serving beef and mushroom pie 1 cup steamed broccoli 8 oz. water
Day	50 grams	8 oz.	1 lean roast	4 whole	1 grilled

| 5 | salmon with 2 scrambled egg ½ medium banana 8 oz. coffee with skim milk and stevia | strawberry and yoghurt crunch 8 oz. water | beef sandwich in barley bread 1 cup steamed broccoli 1 orange 8 oz. water | grain crackers w/ low fat cream cheese 8 oz. water | lamb ½ cup basmati rice 1 cup steamed green beans 8 oz. water |

Recipes

Crab stuffed avocados

Ingredients
- 100g white crabmeat, cooked
- 1 tsp mustard, Dijon
- 2 tbsp. olive oil
- handful basil leaves, shredded with a few of the smaller leaves left whole, to serve
- 1 red chili, deseeded and chopped
- 2 avocados

Instructions
1. Flake the crabmeat in a small bowl. Add the mustard and oil, then mix. Season to taste. Can be prepared a day ahead.
2. Cut the avocadoes in half, remove the stone. Fill each cavity of the avocado with quarter of the crab mixture.
3. Garnish with basil leaf and chili before serving.

Beef Stew

- 1 <u>onion</u>, sliced
- 1 <u>garlic</u> clove, sliced
- 2 tbsp. <u>olive oil</u>
- 300g pack <u>beef</u> stir-fry strips, or use beef steak, thinly sliced
- 1 yellow pepper, deseeded and thinly sliced
- 400g canned chopped <u>tomato</u>
- sprig <u>rosemary</u>, chopped
- handful pitted <u>olives</u>

Instructions

1. In a large saucepan, sauté garlic and onion in olive oil for 5 minutes.
2. Add the beef strips, peppers, tomatoes and rosemary. Simmer for 15 minutes and bring to a boil.
3. Once the meat is cook, add boiling water if needed.
4. Toss the olives and serve with polenta.

Lemon Chicken Salad

Ingredients

- 3/4 cup finely chopped celery
- ¼ cup low-fat mayonnaise
- ¼ cup low-fat plain yogurt
- ¼ cup finely chopped green onions
- 2 tablespoons chopped fresh tarragon
- 3 tablespoons fresh lemon juice
- 1 teaspoon lemon zest
- 3 cooked boneless, skinless chicken breasts, cut into 1/2-inch cubes
- 1 green apple, cored and cut into 1-inch chunks
- Salt and ground black pepper to taste

Instructions

1. In a large bowl, combine the celery, mayonnaise, yogurt, green onions, tarragon, lemon juice and zest and mix thoroughly.
2. Toss in the chicken cubes and apple chunks and fold onto the mixture.
3. Season with salt and pepper before serving.

Grilled Tenderloin

Ingredients

- 4 large garlic cloves, minced
- 2 tablespoons reduced-sodium soy sauce
- 2 teaspoons dried ginger
- 2 teaspoons Dijon mustard
- 1/3 cup fresh lime juice
- 1/3 cup extra-virgin olive oil
- ¼ teaspoon cayenne pepper
- 1 ½ pounds beef tenderloin, well trimmed

Instructions

1. In a large bowl, mix all ingredients except the beef until well blended.
2. Add the beef to the mixture until both sides are coated with the marinade.
3. Marinate in the refrigerator for 8 hours turning the meat halfway through the time to marinate the other side.
4. Take out of the refrigerator and leave in room temperature for 30 minutes before patting it dry.
5. Grill the tenderloin for 22 minutes or until done to your preference.
6. Remove from grill and let it stand for 5 minutes before cutting it crosswise into 1/3-inch strip serving.

Quinoa and Black Beans

Ingredients

- 1 teaspoon vegetable oil
- 1 onion, chopped
- 3 cloves garlic, chopped
- 3/4 cup quinoa
- 1 1/2 cups vegetable broth
- 1 teaspoon ground cumin
- 1/4 teaspoon cayenne pepper
- salt and ground black pepper to taste
- 1 cup frozen corn kernels
- 2 (15 ounce) cans black beans, rinsed and drained
- 1/2 cup chopped fresh cilantro

Instructions

1. In a saucepan over medium heat, cook and stir onion and garlic over heated oil for about 10 minutes.
2. Add quinoa and pour vegetable broth onto the saucepan. Season with cumin, cayenne pepper, salt and black pepper. Bring to a boil.

3. Cover and reduce heat. Simmer for 20 minutes or until quinoa is tender and the broth is fully absorbed.
4. Stir in frozen corn and continue to simmer for about 5 minutes. Add the black beans and cilantro.
5. Serve

Braised Balsamic Chicken

Ingredients

- 6 skinless, boneless chicken breast halves
- 1 teaspoon garlic salt
- ground black pepper to taste
- 2 tablespoons olive oil
- 1 onion, thinly sliced
- 1 (14.5 ounce) can diced tomatoes
- ½ cup balsamic vinegar
- 1 teaspoon dried basil
- 1 teaspoon dried oregano
- 1 teaspoon dried rosemary
- ½ teaspoon dried thyme

Instructions

1. Season the chicken breast with garlic, salt and pepper on all sides.
2. On a skillet over medium heat, heat olive oil and cook each side of the chicken 3 to 4 minutes or until it turns golden brown. Add onion and cook continue to cook for another 4 minutes.
3. Add diced tomatoes and balsamic vinegar. Season with basil, oregano, rosemary and thyme. Check temperature of the pan using a thermometer and see if it reads 165 degrees F (74 degrees C). Cooke the chicken for about 15 minutes or when it is tender.

Tomato and Basil Soup

Ingredients

- 1 medium sized onion
- 1 clove garlic
- 2 tablespoons olive oil
- 8 cherry tomatoes/3 vine tomatoes
- 14oz/400g can plum tomatoes
- 1 teaspoon dried basil or 5 leaves of fresh basil
- ¼ pint/150ml water
- 1 teaspoon salt
- pepper

Instructions

1. Chop onion and tomatoes. Finely slice garlic. Sauté in olive oil onion, tomatoes, garlic, and basil.
2. Add the canned tomatoes, salt and pepper. Cover the pan and let it simmer for 30 minutes on low heat.
3. Transfer to a blender or food processor and blend until smooth.

Chapter 4 Week 3: Evaluation and Adjustments

Time to use your menu plan.
After all the planning and preparation, it's time to put your meal plan into practice.
Week 3

1. Record everything

First thing you need to do is to record all your statistics. Create a record book right on the first day.
Record your weight and your blood sugar count. You need to monitor these two because from these numbers you'll be able to determine if you are getting the results you want.
You will see the effect of the blood sugar count immediately. Take a blood sugar test in the morning before you eat, then take another one after lunch. Compare your blood sugar count and see the difference.
Get another test after your last meal. Record all these on your record book.
Repeat this process daily for the next five days. For diabetics, keeping a record is already part of their daily routine, they only need to continue doing so.

2. Eating according to your meal plan

Do not be complacent.

Observe how your body is reacting to your meal plan. Having food cravings will be normal, as your body needs time to adjust with the changes.

3. Make adjustments on your meal plans

If your blood sugar count is going down, that is good but take note of the speed of decrease. If your sugar is rapidly decreasing, then you need to make adjustments to your meal plan.
The same applies if your blood sugar is increasing or not showing any signs of decreasing.

A non-diabetic person has a normal blood sugar level of 100 mg/dl after fasting for at least eight hours, and less than 140 mg/dl 2 hours after eating.
At daytime, levels are lower just before meals. For non-diabetics, sugar level varies from 60-90 mg/dl.

For diabetics, 70-130 mg/dl before meals is normal and less than 180 mg/dl 2 hours after meals.

Depending on how your body reacts to the meal plan, make the necessary adjustments until you fully acclimatize.

At the end of the 5-day meal plan, check your weight. Low Glycemic Diet is not a weight loss plan so do not expect a huge change there. Any weight loss while under the Low Glycemic Diet is just icing on the cake.

4. Evaluate what works for you

Evaluate your progress. The entire time you are undergoing the exercise, evaluate what works for you.

Try to experiment with other food types. As much as you find it easy to just stick with common types of food, you will get tired of it eventually and you will find yourself leaving the diet.

Don't be afraid to mix and match food groups. As long as you are sticking to the general guideline, then you cannot go wrong.

5. Always keep a record

This is one of the follies of people who are using new eating habits or under a new diet. Keeping a record is important because you would be able to keep track of your progress. It also helps you evaluate what works for you and what won't, thus, you can adjust on the plan.

6. Prepare your next meal plan

You are now ready to prepare your next meal plan. You can choose a weekly meal plan or a 2-week plan.

The longer your plan the cheaper it will be to purchase ingredients. A longer plan will also help keep you stick to it.

Chapter 5 The Last Step: Make it a Habit

The last step in our exercise is how to make the Low Glycemic Diet a habit.

All the planning, the testing and the evaluating will go to waste if you cannot maintain it.
You need to make the low glycemic diet a habit. This is probably the most difficult step in the entire exercise.

Making the Low Glycemic Diet a habit is actually easy because you can still eat the food you like, though there are restrictions.
Here are some tips I'd like to share with you to help you maintain a Low Glycemic Diet.
- Avoid starchy food. Eat leafy greens, beans, and fruits like apple, oranges, peaches, and berries.
- Choose grains. Avoid bread from white flour, instead choose barley, whole wheat, and whole meal choices like sourdough.
- Forget the cereal. Go with the basics like oatmeal, porridge, or natural muesli. If you really cannot go without cereal, choose a brand that has GI stamped on it.
- Choose food groups with healthy fats like olive oil, nuts (walnuts, almonds, pecans), and avocado but keep it moderate.

- Limit sweets like ice cream and fruit juices.
- Eat foods rich in protein like meat, fish, seafood and poultry but keep it moderate.
- Acid can slow down conversion of carbohydrates into sugar. Food with high acid content like sourdough, oranges, vinaigrette have low glycemic count.
- Cook food have higher glycemic index value than uncooked foods.

Dining Out

Eating out is usually a nightmare for people who are on a diet. You have no control over the food that is served. You can probably go to vegan restaurants but if your companions are not vegan, you don't have much of a choice. Many restaurants nowadays are offering a variety of healthy foods. It is just a matter of choosing the right kind of food to order.
If you are dining out, it is safer to go in a restaurant than a fast food chain. Avoid fast food because every food they have are high in glycemic count.

Conclusion

I'd like to thank you and congratulate you for taking this journey with me from start to finish. I hope this book was able to help you to learn more about Low Glycemic Index and its benefits. I hope you also enjoyed doing the sample exercise with me.

The next step is making the Low Glycemic Diet your new healthy habit. It is not really a big step to take. You just need to shift your gears and start making smart choices.

Do not count the calories; count the glycemic value so you can start living clean and healthy.

I wish you the best of luck!

mindplusfood

THANK YOU FOR YOUR PURCHASE

VISIT MINDPLUSFOOD.COM FOR A
FREE 41-PAGE HOLISTIC HEALTH
CHEAT SHEET

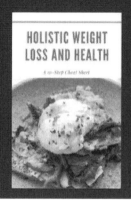

Printed in Great Britain
by Amazon